© Laura McGregor
First Published: 2024

Paperback ISBN: 9798346141013

Healing for the Holidays

A Cancer Survivor's Inspiring Christmas Diary

Laura McGregor

Dedication

To my beloved husband, Albert, whose love and unwavering support were the pillars that held me up when I thought I could fall no further.

To my children, Linda, Margaret, and Jimmy, whose laughter, compassion, and joy have been the light in the darkest of times.

And to all the cancer fighters, survivors, and their families, who carry the strength of hope and the courage to keep fighting, even when the path seems impossible.

This book is for you—may it remind you that healing is possible, and that love, faith, and resilience are the greatest forces we possess.

Acknowledgements

This book would not have been possible without the love, support, and guidance of so many people who stood by me during one of the most difficult chapters of my life. I am deeply grateful for each and every person who contributed to my journey, and I wish to take this moment to acknowledge their unwavering strength and love.

First, I owe everything to my family. To my husband, Albert, whose strength, patience, and undying love carried me through the darkest days. Your constant presence and belief in me were the anchor I needed when the storm seemed too strong to weather. Thank you for never letting me go, for always reminding me that hope was still alive, and for loving me with a heart so pure. You are the foundation of my healing.

To my children—Linda, Margaret, and Jimmy—your love and laughter were the rays of sunshine I desperately needed. Linda, your wisdom and compassion, far beyond your years, gave me the courage to keep moving forward. Margaret, your infectious smile and unrelenting support reminded me daily that there is joy even in the midst of sorrow. Jimmy, your innocence and energy filled our home with light and reminded me to find joy in the small moments. You three kept me grounded, and your love nourished me when I thought I had nothing left.

To my extended family, friends, and loved ones, thank you for offering your prayers, your kind words, and your comforting presence. Even when I couldn't fully articulate what I was going through, you all knew how to show up. I am deeply blessed to have you in my life.

A special thank you to the alternative therapist who opened my eyes to a new world of healing. Your knowledge, your gentle encouragement, and your belief in the power of nature were instrumental in my recovery. You gave me the tools to heal not just my body, but my soul. The journey would not have been the same without your wisdom.

To all the healthcare professionals who cared for me—doctors, nurses, and therapists—you provided me with the best medical care, and I am thankful for your dedication. While orthodox treatments were only one part of my healing journey, I respect and honor your expertise and commitment to improving lives.

I am profoundly grateful for the healing communities and spiritual centers I visited. Your warmth, compassion, and prayers were a constant source of strength, and you reminded me that faith and hope are just as essential as medicine. Your unwavering belief in miracles brought comfort during my most trying times, and I carry those teachings with me.

I also want to express my gratitude to all the cancer fighters and survivors I met along the way. Our shared experiences, strength, and support created a bond that I will forever cherish. You are my inspiration and my reminder that we are all in this together. Your stories of perseverance, resilience, and courage kept me going even when my own will faltered.

To the countless herbalists and alternative healers who share their wisdom with the world: you gave me a new understanding of how the earth offers us the tools we need to heal. I am so grateful for your dedication to preserving ancient healing traditions and for the hope you've restored in me.

Finally, to you, the reader, thank you for picking up this book. I hope my story touches you in a way that helps you on your own journey, whether you are dealing with cancer, a personal struggle, or simply searching for hope. Writing this book has been my way of giving back, and if it brings even a moment of light or relief to someone, then it has been worth every word.

I have come to learn that healing is not a solitary journey—it is one that we take together, supported by the love and care of those around us. This book is a testament to that truth, and I dedicate it to all the people who have ever touched my life and helped me heal.

With all my love and gratitude,
Laura McGregor

Contents

Afterword 139

Preface

Life has a way of surprising us, of throwing us into the unknown, and challenging our very essence. Sometimes, it's a gentle nudge, a fleeting moment that asks us to step out of our comfort zone. Other times, it's an overwhelming storm that leaves us questioning everything we thought we knew about ourselves, about the world, and about what we are capable of enduring.

For me, it was cancer.

But my journey through cancer was not just a battle with a disease; it was a confrontation with every part of my life—my body, my mind, my spirit, and the way I understood what it means to heal. It was a path paved with pain, uncertainty, and deep moments of despair. But it was also a journey of unexpected discoveries, of moments of grace, and most importantly, it was a journey toward **hope**.

I wasn't supposed to make it. At least, that's what my diagnosis told me. The doctors, the treatments, the medications—they all promised the same thing: you'll have to endure, you'll have to fight. But no one really prepared me for the other battle—the battle for my **soul**. The one where you wake up in the morning and wonder if the pain will ever subside, or if the tears will ever stop falling. The battle that questions your worth, your strength, and your belief in yourself. This was the fight that often felt like the hardest one to win.

But somehow, despite it all, I found my way through.

I began to realize that healing doesn't always come in the form of a pill, a doctor's order, or a prayer in a church. Sometimes, healing comes in the form of a **shift**—a shift in mindset, in belief, in how we view ourselves and the world. For me, that shift came when I opened my mind to alternatives—both in medicine and in how I approached life itself. It was in that shift that I found healing. It was in the unlikeliest of places, in the form of natural remedies, ancient wisdom, and the unwavering belief that my body had the **capacity** to heal itself, if only I would give it the right tools, the right love, and the right **patience**.

This book is my story—a story of pain, yes, but more than that, it's a story of transformation. It's the story of how I moved from the deepest despair to the highest joy, how I learned to **trust** again, how I discovered the power of **herbs** and healing, and how I found strength in the love and support of those around me. It's a story of **laughter** in the face of hardship, of joy in the midst of suffering, and of triumph in the most unlikely of circumstances.

The pages that follow are not just for those who are fighting cancer. They are for anyone who has ever felt like giving up, anyone who has ever felt like the weight of the world was too heavy to bear. They are for those who are in the middle of their own battle—whether it's an illness, a loss, or any challenge that life has thrown their way. I hope that through my words, you find comfort, you find strength, and you find the courage to keep moving forward, no matter how difficult the path may seem.

This book is about resilience—about the ability to rise when you feel like you're being buried. It's about **hope**—about never giving up, even when the odds are stacked against you.

It's about **love**—the kind of love that doesn't just heal wounds but lifts you up when you're too weak to stand on your own. It's about **joy**—the joy that comes when you discover, against all odds, that you can still experience happiness, laughter, and peace, even in the most trying of times.

I want to invite you into my world—into my battle, my healing, and my ultimate **victory**. This book is a testament to the fact that no matter what you're facing, there is always hope, and there is always a way through the darkness to the light on the other side. I'm not here to tell you that the journey is easy, or that the road is without pain. But I am here to tell you that it is **worth it**. That no matter how difficult it may seem, you are not alone. You are **stronger** than you think. And you **can** heal.

So, welcome. Welcome to my story. Welcome to the journey of healing, of hope, and of finding your way through the storm. May these pages offer you not just words, but a light that guides you when you feel lost, a hope that lifts you when you feel down, and a reminder that you are never, ever alone.

With love,
Laura McGregor

Chapter 1: The Darkest Hour

The Diagnosis

I remember the day like it was yesterday. The cold, sterile walls of the doctor's office felt like they were closing in, amplifying every nervous breath, every tremor of my hand. My name—Laura McGregor—was called with a kind but firm voice that I now associate with the piercing pain of reality. I had come in for a routine check-up, expecting to be out in a matter of minutes, perhaps with a quick reminder to drink more water or cut back on caffeine. But life had other plans.

When the doctor started talking, I noticed the tone in his voice was different, cautious yet compassionate. He hesitated, glancing at my husband, Albert, before uttering the words: "Laura, you have cervical cancer." I froze. In that moment, everything felt surreal, like I was watching someone else's life unfold on a screen. Cancer wasn't supposed to happen to me. I was a mother of three—Linda, a bright 19-year-old undergraduate; Margaret, my sweet 15-year-old high schooler; and little Jimmy, only seven years old, just beginning his journey in the world. This couldn't be my reality.

The room seemed to fade as waves of questions and fears washed over me. How would my family manage? Who would look after the kids if something happened to me? Would I even get to see Jimmy grow up, walk Linda down the aisle, or watch Margaret blossom into her dreams? My mind was consumed with these fears, yet I struggled to hold it together for Albert, who squeezed my hand, silently offering strength even as I could see the dread in his eyes.

The days following the diagnosis were a blur. I alternated between feeling numb and breaking down, unable to hold back the tears that would come unbidden, even at the smallest trigger. I felt as though a shadow had fallen over my life, one that I couldn't escape no matter how hard I tried. My days became a haze of doctor's visits, test results, and discussions about treatment options. Each conversation brought new terms and realities I had to absorb—stages, survival rates, chemotherapy. These words took on a dreadful, almost sinister quality in my mind.

Yet, I also felt a strange pressure to hide my true feelings. I wanted to protect my children from the reality that their mother was facing something as terrifying as cancer. When Linda came home from college and asked if everything was all right, I found myself plastering on a smile, swallowing back the lump in my throat as I assured her that everything would be fine. For Margaret, I made extra efforts to listen to her teenage worries, hoping my calm presence would mask my inner turmoil. And with Jimmy, I took extra time to play and laugh, his innocent joy giving me a reprieve from the darkness within me.

However, at night, alone in bed with Albert, I would let the facade crumble. In those quiet hours, he held me as I cried, as I voiced my deepest fears—what if I wasn't strong enough to endure this? What if I never made it out on the other side? Albert would listen patiently, his rough hands wiping away my tears, whispering words of encouragement, and praying aloud for strength and healing. Through his unwavering support, I realized that I didn't have to face this alone.

Searching for Strength

As the days turned into weeks, I sought strength from sources I had once taken for granted. Faith, which had been a quiet part of my life, now became my anchor. I began praying like never before, often pleading with God in the quiet moments of the day to grant me the strength I needed, if not for myself, then for my children and Albert. I found comfort in attending church services and meeting with the pastor, who offered words of encouragement and even connected me with other cancer survivors in our congregation. Their stories of survival filled me with hope that perhaps, just perhaps, I could be one of the fortunate ones.

I leaned heavily on the love of my family. My daughters, who quickly sensed that something was amiss, showed an unexpected maturity that both broke and healed my heart. Linda took on extra responsibilities at home and even postponed a few social plans, assuring me that her place was by my side. Margaret, though young, offered a gentle comfort that I will never forget. She left little notes by my bedside, each one a reminder of her love and belief in me, and would often spend her evenings curled up by my side, just holding my hand in silence.

Albert, my rock, continued to be my strongest support. Even as he shouldered the financial burden and worked long hours, he would come home and insist on handling household tasks to allow me the rest I so desperately needed. There were moments of laughter amid the pain, moments where Albert's humor—simple jokes or lighthearted stories from his day at the docks—would bring a smile to my face. It was in these moments that I realized how deeply I was loved and how much strength that love gave me.

As I stood on the brink of this uncertain journey, I knew one thing with absolute clarity: I could not do this alone. My family was my reason for fighting, my reason for hoping that someday, I would look back on this period as a dark chapter that eventually led to a beautiful rebirth. And in the deepest recesses of my heart, I clung to a vision—a vision of sitting by a beautifully lit Christmas tree, surrounded by my children and Albert, sharing laughter and stories, and reveling in the simple joy of being alive. It was this image that kept me going, this hope of a future filled with love and light.

Chapter 2: Trials of Treatment

Chemo and Pain

The first round of chemotherapy was like stepping into the unknown. I had heard stories from others about the horrors of chemo, but I hadn't fully understood what it would mean to experience it firsthand. Sitting in the sterile hospital room with an IV line in my arm, watching the clear liquid slowly drip into my veins, I felt a strange combination of hope and dread. This was supposed to help me—this toxic potion that I was willingly letting into my body was supposed to fight the cancer cells, to give me a chance at more years with my family. But as the nurse adjusted the flow and gave me a sympathetic smile, I couldn't shake the gnawing fear that I was poisoning myself, all in the name of survival.

The days following that first session were like a descent into a physical and emotional abyss. The nausea hit me with a force I couldn't have imagined. I couldn't hold down food or water, my body rejecting even the simplest meals. Every smell turned my stomach, every taste felt like metal, and I was left feeling weak and frail. My bones ached as though they were being twisted from the inside, and every muscle screamed with exhaustion even after the shortest movement. Sleep, once my escape from fear, became a cruel and shallow refuge. I would lie awake for hours, every twinge of pain reminding me of the cancer lurking inside me, and the punishing treatment that was supposed to save me.

One evening, as I lay curled up on the bathroom floor, overcome by another wave of nausea, Jimmy tiptoed in and sat down beside me. He was too young to understand the full scope of my illness, but he knew I was hurting. Quietly, he placed his small hand on mine, his innocent eyes filled with concern. "Are you going to be okay, Mommy?" he asked softly. I mustered a weak smile, swallowing back the lump in my throat, and nodded, reassuring him even though I didn't feel certain myself. That night, as I watched him drift off to sleep, I promised myself that I would do everything in my power to keep fighting. For Jimmy. For Linda and Margaret. For Albert. For all of them.

Feeling Trapped

As the chemo sessions continued, I found myself sinking deeper into a sense of isolation. My body became a stranger to me, a vessel of pain and sickness that I no longer recognized. My hair began to fall out in clumps, a tangible reminder of the war waging inside my body.

One morning, as I watched the strands collect in the sink, I broke down, the tears flowing freely. I hadn't realized how much my hair had been a part of my identity until I saw it slipping away. I felt stripped, exposed, like every part of me was being taken by this disease.

The changes weren't just physical. I felt a distance growing between myself and the world outside. Friends who once called regularly began to drift away, their voices hesitant, unsure of what to say. Even well-meaning comments sometimes stung. "Stay positive," they'd urge, or "You're strong—you'll beat this." They didn't see the nights where I lay awake, feeling weak and frightened, too drained to even pray. I felt like I was in a prison of my own body, bound by pain and exhaustion, unable to escape. I missed the Laura I used to be—the energetic mom, the loving wife, the woman who faced life with a laugh and a smile. Now, it seemed like every ounce of energy I had was focused solely on survival.

Albert, though, never wavered. He continued to be my lifeline, my anchor. Every morning, he would sit by my bedside before leaving for work, his rough hands gently brushing back the few strands of hair that remained. "You're beautiful, Laura," he'd say softly, his eyes full of love. I wanted to believe him, wanted to see the beauty he claimed was still there. But the mirror showed a different story—a woman pale and gaunt, her skin stretched tight over her bones, her eyes hollow and haunted. I felt trapped inside this new version of myself, yearning for the day I could break free.

A Family's Support

Despite the isolation, my family became my source of light in those darkest days. Each of them, in their own way, found ways to lift my spirits, to remind me that I was not alone in this battle. Linda, balancing her studies with the heavy weight of worry, would bring me books, hoping the familiar comfort of words would distract me. She'd curl up beside me, reading aloud when my strength failed, her voice a soothing balm on my raw nerves. She would often end her readings with stories of her day, weaving in the humor and small victories that filled her life. Through her words, I felt a glimmer of the life outside my hospital bed—a life I desperately wanted to return to.

Margaret took on more responsibilities around the house, her youthful spirit undeterred by the weight she now carried. I watched in awe as she helped with Jimmy, keeping him entertained with games and stories, often making him laugh with her dramatic reenactments of their favorite shows. When Margaret wasn't with Jimmy, she would sit by my side, filling the room with her art supplies, painting and drawing with a focus that seemed to channel the worries we all felt. She would hand me her drawings, pictures of sunflowers, of smiling families, of starry skies—a reminder of the beauty that still existed beyond my pain.

And Jimmy, my sweet boy, with his innocent joy, became my greatest comfort. He would climb onto my lap, resting his head on my chest, his small hands tracing the lines of my face as though memorizing every detail. "Mommy," he would say in his quiet, serious way, "when you get better, can we go to the zoo again?" His faith in my recovery, unshakable in his young mind, became a source of strength. I would nod, brushing my fingers through his hair, making promises I wasn't sure I could keep, but knowing that, in that moment, they gave me hope.

Albert's love remained steadfast. He took on the role of caregiver with a gentle strength that left me in awe. He would cook when he could, sometimes bringing me small meals I could stomach, his every action filled with care. One evening, as I sat quietly by the fire, wrapped in a blanket to keep the chills at bay, he shared stories from his day at the docks, recounting funny incidents and mishaps. He even tried to make me laugh, reenacting a slip he'd had that nearly sent him tumbling into the water. I laughed, the sound foreign yet welcome, a small reminder of the woman I used to be.

Together, we found moments of humor and joy, even amidst the overwhelming pain. The love my family poured into me became the fuel that kept me going. Their presence reminded me that this battle was not mine alone, and that every day I held on was a victory for all of us. As I faced each trial, each wave of pain, I clung to the warmth of their love, knowing that they were my reason for enduring, my hope for the future, and my light in the darkness.

Chapter 3: In Search of Miracles

Prayers in the Dark

In the darkest moments, I turned to prayer with a desperate fervor. It wasn't a new habit—I'd prayed for years, asking for protection over my family, for guidance in difficult times, for blessings upon our lives. But now, my prayers took on a raw, urgent quality as I pleaded for my own life, asking for strength, for healing, and sometimes, in my most vulnerable moments, simply for relief from the pain. I felt I was no longer speaking to God in calm, reverent tones; rather, I was crying out with an intensity that came from the depths of my suffering. Alone in my room, clutching the edges of my blanket, I would whisper every word, as if speaking quietly might somehow make my prayers more powerful, more likely to reach the heavens.

There were nights when my faith faltered, when I wondered if God was listening at all. Why would He allow me, a wife, a mother, a woman who loved her family and did her best to be kind to others, to suffer this way? I questioned, I doubted, and yet, I couldn't bring myself to abandon the act of praying. Each time I closed my eyes, I imagined a light in the darkness, a glimmer of hope that perhaps God had a plan, one I couldn't yet understand. I found myself returning to certain verses, repeating them like mantras. "The Lord is my shepherd; I shall not want..." I would whisper, feeling the words anchor me, holding me steady as the pain surged and ebbed.

My family, too, embraced prayer as a means of supporting me. Albert would kneel beside my bed each night, his hands clasped tightly, his head bowed in silent concentration. Even though he wasn't a deeply religious man, he prayed with a devotion that brought tears to my eyes. Sometimes, Linda and Margaret would join him, their soft voices filling the room as they took turns asking for my healing, their words filled with love and hope. Jimmy, my youngest, would clasp his small hands together, his voice a soft whisper as he said, "Please make Mommy better." Each of them carried their faith like a torch, illuminating the path forward even when it felt unbearably dark.

In my conversations with God, I tried to find meaning in my suffering, searching for answers that could help me endure. There were moments when I felt a strange calm wash over me, as though a quiet voice within was telling me to hold on, to keep believing that relief would come. Yet, there were also nights when the pain seemed endless, and I was convinced that my prayers had been lost, floating somewhere in the void, unheard and unanswered.

One day, Linda brought home a small, white candle, which she placed on my nightstand. "It's a prayer candle, Mom," she explained, her eyes bright with optimism. "They say that lighting it while you pray can bring comfort and healing." We lit the candle together, watching the tiny flame flicker to life, its warm glow casting gentle shadows around the room. From that day on, each night as I prayed, I would light the candle, letting its light soothe me, a symbol of my faith in the possibility of healing. And though my journey through prayer was filled with doubt, hope, despair, and moments of peace, that candle remained my constant companion, a quiet reminder that even in the darkness, there was always light.

Desperate for relief, I found myself exploring every avenue that might offer healing, including visits to various miracle centers. These centers were scattered across cities and towns, each one known for its healing services, miraculous testimonies, and charismatic healers. Some were quiet, small rooms filled with prayer, while others were grand auditoriums echoing with songs, prayers, and cries for healing. These places were filled with people just like me—mothers, fathers, children, all seeking the same miracle, the same touch of divine intervention that might free us from our pain.

Albert drove me to the first center, a modest building with a simple sign: "Healing Hands Ministry." The moment we stepped inside, we were greeted by the smell of incense and the low murmur of prayers. People sat in rows, heads bowed, some with tears streaming down their faces, others holding their loved ones' hands tightly. The atmosphere was thick with desperation and hope, the air charged with the collective belief that miracles were not just possible but real. I watched as the healer, a tall, solemn man, moved among the crowd, touching people's foreheads, whispering words of blessing, his hands trembling with what he claimed was the power of God.

When he reached me, he placed his hand gently on my shoulder and closed his eyes, murmuring a prayer. I closed my own eyes, trying to focus on his words, to absorb every syllable as if it were medicine. "In the name of Jesus," he whispered, his voice soft but powerful, "I command this sickness to leave. I command healing to flow through this body." I felt a warmth spread through me, a tingling sensation that filled me with a strange hope. But as we left that center, the pain returned, stubbornly persistent, reminding me that the path to healing was not as simple as a single touch.

Our journey took us to several more centers, each offering a unique approach to healing. Some practiced anointing with oils, the healers pouring fragrant oils over my head, my hands, my shoulders, their voices filled with conviction as they prayed for my recovery. Others relied on song and dance, encouraging the sick to rise, to clap and move as a way of inviting healing into their lives. I participated, lifting my hands, moving as much as my weakened body allowed, trying to summon the energy to believe in a miracle.

There were moments in these centers when I felt genuine hope, a spark of something that seemed like healing energy flowing through me. But each time, the pain would return, often stronger than before, leaving me feeling more broken than I had been.

I began to wonder if I was wrong for seeking these places, for hoping that a single touch, a prayer, or a dance could cure something as complex as cancer. And yet, with each visit, I felt a renewed determination. These experiences, though they did not bring the miracle I sought, reminded me of the power of hope, of belief, of the community of others who shared my suffering.

In those days, my faith was both my anchor and my burden. I clung to it because it was all I had, but at times, I felt as though I was carrying a weight that grew heavier with each passing day. I wrestled with my beliefs, questioning everything I thought I knew about God, about suffering, about the nature of miracles. It was a struggle that often left me feeling conflicted—one moment filled with hope, the next consumed by despair.

I sought solace in scripture, reading verses that spoke of God's love and mercy, of His ability to heal the sick, to raise the dead, to make the impossible possible. Yet, with each passage I read, I couldn't help but feel a growing frustration. If God had performed miracles in the past, if He was truly capable of healing, then why was I still suffering? Why did my prayers feel like they were falling on deaf ears? The more I read, the more I questioned, until I found myself on the edge of abandoning my faith entirely.

But then, in moments of clarity, I would remember the times when I had felt something beyond myself—a gentle, comforting presence, a quiet assurance that I was not alone. These glimpses of peace were fleeting, but they gave me a sense of purpose, a reminder that even though I was in pain, my journey had meaning. I wasn't sure what that meaning was, but I held on to the hope that one day I would understand.

My struggle with faith became a journey in itself, a path lined with doubts, fears, and small revelations. I learned to accept that faith wasn't about having all the answers, but about finding strength in the face of uncertainty. In those moments of prayer, in the quiet of the night, I made peace with the fact that I might never know why I was chosen to walk this path. But as long as I had the love of my family, the support of those around me, and the faintest spark of belief, I would keep going, one day at a time.

Chapter 4: The Lowest Point

Depression and Suicidal Thoughts

Cancer had brought with it a shadow that clung to me—a weight that was as heavy on my spirit as it was on my body. The physical pain was only part of the battle; the toll on my mental health became a war of its own. I had once been a person filled with laughter, joy, and endless hope, but now, I often felt like a hollow version of myself, just going through the motions. Each day, as I struggled to get out of bed, I found myself trapped in a cycle of despair, sinking deeper into a pit that seemed to have no bottom.

The relentless pain and the frustration of treatments that seemed to bring no relief pushed me into a depression unlike anything I'd ever known. I would sit in silence for hours, staring out the window, watching the world go by as if I were no longer a part of it. My children would try to cheer me up with their little jokes and stories, and my husband, Albert, was always by my side, gently coaxing me to smile or eat something. But there were days when I simply couldn't find the energy to respond. I felt like a burden, a shadow that brought only worry to those I loved most.

At my lowest point, thoughts of ending the suffering began to creep into my mind. I'd never imagined myself considering such a thing; the thought alone terrified me. But there were moments when it seemed like the only escape, a way to end the pain, the endless cycle of hope and disappointment. I would lie awake at night, haunted by the image of my own absence and the strange peace I imagined might come with it. Yet, even in those dark hours, I was gripped by an overwhelming sense of guilt. How could I leave behind my children, my husband, the people who had done so much to support me? It was a toxic cycle—feeling like a burden, then feeling guilty for even thinking about leaving them with such a loss.

The nights were the hardest. In the darkness, I felt most vulnerable, my thoughts taking on a life of their own, filling my mind with questions, doubts, and fears that seemed impossible to silence. Sometimes, I would wander through the house, moving from room to room, trying to find a place where I could escape the feelings that had become all too familiar. I was searching for peace, but it felt like a distant memory, something I could no longer reach. And as much as I tried to shake myself out of it, the depression only tightened its grip, leaving me feeling powerless, adrift in a sea of hopelessness.

Looking back now, I realize that those moments were perhaps the most dangerous, the times when I was closest to surrendering. The experience of facing my mortality in such a profound way was terrifying, yet it was also a reminder of how fragile our mental health can be, especially when faced with something as overwhelming as cancer. It was in those dark, quiet hours that I began to understand the importance of reaching out, of not allowing myself to be alone with my thoughts for too long. Though I didn't know it yet, this realization would eventually become the turning point in my battle against both the disease and the depression that came with it.

My struggles weren't only with the illness and my depression, but with an intense sense of guilt that I carried daily. As a mother and wife, I had always felt a deep responsibility to care for my family, to be their rock, the one they could rely on for comfort and stability. Now, it felt like I had failed them. Instead of being a source of joy and support, I felt like a burden—someone they had to look after, someone who needed their constant attention. Watching my family care for me with worried faces and quiet conversations was almost as painful as the illness itself.

The guilt I felt was overwhelming. Linda and Margaret, my daughters, were both in important phases of their lives—Linda in college, Margaret navigating high school. These were supposed to be exciting, carefree years for them, and yet, they were weighed down by their mother's illness. They would come home with stories of their day, only to find me too weak or too distracted by pain to listen. It broke my heart each time I saw the disappointment in their eyes, the way they would catch themselves mid-sentence, as if remembering that I wasn't the same mother they used to know.

Albert, my husband, was perhaps the one who suffered the most. He had always been my partner, my equal, someone I could lean on in difficult times. But now, he had taken on the role of caregiver, a responsibility that required patience, resilience, and strength that seemed unfair to place on him. I knew he was exhausted from long hours at the dock, yet every evening, he would come home, set aside his own needs, and tend to mine. I would watch him from across the room, his face lined with worry and fatigue, and the guilt would tighten around my heart. I felt as though I had stolen the life we had planned together, replacing it with a reality filled with hospital visits, medications, and a constant state of uncertainty.

Even Jimmy, my youngest, bore the weight of my illness in ways I hadn't anticipated. He was only seven, a child who should have been carefree, his world filled with play and laughter. Instead, he would come to my bedside, his little face filled with a seriousness that seemed too mature for his years. "Mommy, are you feeling better?" he would ask, his voice filled with a hopeful innocence that made me feel both touched and heartbroken. I wanted so desperately to reassure him, to tell him that everything would be fine, but I knew that words alone couldn't change the reality we were living.

The guilt consumed me, leaving me feeling as though I had let everyone down. I was caught in a web of self-blame, unable to escape the belief that I was somehow responsible for the suffering my family was enduring. I tried to remind myself that cancer was not something I had chosen, that it was not my fault. But these rational thoughts were often drowned out by the intense emotions that came with watching my loved ones struggle alongside me. It was a burden I carried alone, a silent weight that grew heavier with each passing day.

Love that Saved Me

In my lowest moments, when the depression and guilt seemed almost too much to bear, it was the love of my family that ultimately pulled me back from the brink. Each member of my family, in their own way, reminded me that I was not alone, that I was surrounded by a love so strong that it could withstand even the darkest times. Their love became my lifeline, a thread that held me steady as I navigated the churning waters of illness and despair.

Albert, with his quiet, unwavering presence, was my rock. He didn't always have the words to comfort me, but he didn't need them. He showed his love in the way he sat by my side, holding my hand, offering me silent strength. He took on the daily burdens of life without complaint, allowing me the space to focus on my recovery. In his eyes, I saw a commitment that went beyond words, a devotion that told me that no matter how difficult things became, he would be there.

Linda and Margaret, my daughters, found ways to bring light into my days, filling our home with laughter and love even when the atmosphere felt heavy. They would sit beside me, telling me stories of their day, their voices filled with enthusiasm, their laughter like music. They brought me books to read, games to play, and sometimes, they would simply sit with me in silence, their presence a reminder that I was not alone in my struggle. Their love gave me the courage to keep fighting, to believe that there was still joy to be found, even in the midst of suffering.

And then there was Jimmy, my little boy, who reminded me of the simple beauty of a child's love. He would bring me his favorite toys, insisting that they would make me feel better, his innocent gestures filling my heart with a warmth that no medicine could provide. His love was pure, untainted by fear or worry, a reminder of the goodness in life, even when things seemed bleak.

In the end, it was their love that saved me. They reminded me that my life was not just my own, that it was intertwined with theirs, that my presence mattered in ways I hadn't fully realized. Their love gave me a reason to keep going, to keep fighting, to hold on to hope. It became my anchor, grounding me in a reality that was filled with both pain and beauty. And as I held onto that love, I began to find a strength within myself that I had thought was lost—a strength that would carry me forward, through the darkest nights and into the light of a new dawn.

Chapter 5: The Alternative Path

After months of battling through conventional treatments—each chemotherapy session stripping away not only my energy but also my spirit—I began to question if traditional medicine was the only option. My body and mind craved something gentler, something that wouldn't drain my energy to the point of collapse. I realized it was time to consider a different path, yet I struggled with how to take that first step. What could this new path look like, and would it offer real hope?

As I explored my options, I connected with cancer survivors who had taken alternative routes. Their stories were captivating. Many spoke of dietary changes, adopting plant-based diets or fasting practices to detoxify the body.

Others swore by meditation, prayer, and visualization as ways to calm the mind and allow the body to focus on healing. These testimonials painted a picture of people not merely surviving but thriving, their vitality and optimism reignited by their alternative approaches.

One evening, while scrolling through an online support group, I found the story of a woman who had not only survived but flourished by incorporating *Cannabis sativa* and *Cannabidiol* (CBD) into her regimen. Her journey mirrored my own in many ways: endless cycles of chemotherapy, trips to the emergency room, and a profound sense of fatigue. But unlike me, she had found a turning point in alternative medicine, using these natural compounds to regain control over her health. She spoke about the pain relief, the anti-inflammatory effects, and the way her mental clarity improved over time. Her testimony was unlike anything I had read before.

Her story planted a seed in my mind, one that grew with each passing day. I knew I needed a different approach, and with each new piece of information I found on *Cannabis sativa* and CBD, I felt that this was the path calling to me. This discovery didn't erase my doubts—questions swirled in my mind about its effectiveness and safety. But with every story, every patient experience, and every bit of research, my conviction grew stronger. Finally, I knew it was time to try a new path, and this path involved embracing nature's own medicine.

The Role of Herbal Therapy

When I committed to exploring alternative treatments, I found myself introduced to a therapist who specialized in herbal and plant-based therapies, including the use of *Cannabis sativa* and *CBD*. He was a calm and empathetic figure who had a deep understanding of herbal medicine and its role in supporting healing. He explained that *Cannabis sativa* was not about achieving quick cures or miracle results; rather, it was about working in tandem with the body's own healing mechanisms, providing relief, and restoring balance.

The therapist began by explaining the benefits of *Cannabis sativa* and *CBD*. Unlike traditional painkillers, *CBD*, a non-psychoactive compound derived from the cannabis plant, offers significant pain relief without inducing any "high." This was important to me, as I wanted to maintain a clear mind while managing the persistent aches and pains that had become a part of my daily life. The therapist's approach was gradual and cautious, beginning with low doses of *CBD* oil to observe how my body responded. The results were nothing short of astounding. Within days, I felt a reduction in pain, and my joints, which had been stiff and aching, began to relax. It was as though my body had found an ally, a natural relief that allowed me to feel like myself again.

Cannabis sativa, known for its anti-inflammatory properties, also played a crucial role in my healing. Alongside *CBD*, it helped to minimize inflammation and improve my immune response. Unlike the harsh effects of chemotherapy, this herbal therapy worked in harmony with my body, giving me relief without the accompanying exhaustion. I soon began to appreciate how each component of the plant served a specific purpose. The anti-anxiety effects of *CBD* brought a calmness I hadn't felt in months, easing the emotional weight of my journey.

Additionally, my therapist suggested other herbs to complement the *Cannabis sativa*, including ones that supported digestion and overall immune strength. My body started to feel like a thriving ecosystem rather than a battlefield, a place where I was not constantly at war but rather in the process of nurturing back to health. Through herbal therapy, I found that healing was not just about attacking the illness; it was about nourishing the entire body, providing it with the tools to rebuild.

With each passing day, I grew stronger. The pain was still present, but it no longer held dominion over my life. Herbal therapy, especially the potent combination of *Cannabis sativa* and *CBD*, gave me relief that conventional medicine hadn't been able to provide. It reminded me of the power of nature's medicine, teaching me that healing could come not from forcing my body to comply but from supporting it to recover.

Believing in a New Way

Choosing alternative therapies meant reshaping my entire belief system around healing. I had been trained to trust doctors, to believe in hospitals and pharmaceutical treatments. Turning my faith toward *Cannabis sativa* and *CBD* felt like stepping onto foreign soil, unfamiliar but filled with the promise of something new and life-giving. This leap required not only faith in the plants but also trust in myself and in my ability to discern what my body needed.

There were moments of doubt—days when the pain flared up unexpectedly, and my resolve wavered. Friends and family members expressed their concern, worried about my choice to step outside of mainstream treatments. But as my body continued to respond, as the pain subsided and I could finally breathe without wincing, I knew that this path was the right one for me. Every success story, every day of reduced pain, reinforced my belief in the power of nature and the body's innate capacity to heal when given the right support.

One of the biggest transformations was my mindset. *Cannabis sativa* and *CBD* offered not only physical relief but a mental shift, helping to calm my racing thoughts and alleviate the constant anxiety I had about my future. I learned to appreciate each day for the small victories it held, to take comfort in the progress I was making rather than focusing solely on reaching an endpoint. I found peace in the present moment, in the process of healing rather than an imagined destination of "cured."

I realized that healing wasn't about erasing my cancer; it was about restoring harmony and joy to my life. My alternative therapy journey taught me to view my body as a partner, not an enemy to be conquered. With every dose of CBD oil, every herbal tea, I was investing in a future that was rooted not in fear but in love, resilience, and faith.

Embracing this new way of healing required me to release my old expectations and to open my heart to possibilities beyond the boundaries of traditional medicine. *Cannabis sativa* and CBD became symbols of that transformation, tools that allowed me to believe not only in their power but in my own. With each passing day, I grew more committed to this path, finding strength in my ability to forge a life that was vibrant, fulfilling, and entirely my own.

Chapter 6: Steps to Healing

Embarking on a healing journey with alternative treatments introduced me to a new framework of daily choices, a delicate balance of do's and don'ts that became the foundation of my approach to health. The therapist I worked with emphasized that a successful healing path required both commitment and consistency. This process wasn't just about following a protocol; it was about adopting a lifestyle that supported and honored my body's needs, an approach rooted in respect, patience, and trust.

One of the primary "do's" was hydration. Water became a central component of my routine, as it was essential in flushing out toxins and ensuring my body could properly process the herbs and nutrients I was incorporating. I learned to drink water with intention, adding slices of lemon or a sprinkle of sea salt to aid absorption and provide minerals. This seemingly simple act of drinking water became a ritual, a small but meaningful step toward rehydrating my cells and replenishing my system.

Nutrition was another area with essential "do's" and "don'ts." My therapist recommended a diet high in fresh vegetables, whole grains, and lean proteins, while advising me to avoid processed foods, refined sugars, and excessive salt, as they could contribute to inflammation and weaken the immune system. Green leafy vegetables, particularly kale, spinach, and Swiss chard, were rich in antioxidants and phytonutrients that supported cellular repair. Incorporating these foods into my diet allowed me to feel nourished and energized rather than weighed down or sluggish.

However, diet wasn't only about what to eat but also what to avoid. Processed foods, for instance, were strictly off-limits. I had to remove foods that contained artificial additives, preservatives, and unhealthy fats, as these could hinder my progress and compromise the efficacy of the herbs I was taking. While initially, this was challenging—especially during gatherings where processed and sugary foods were common—the discipline gradually transformed my relationship with food. I began to see each meal as an opportunity to heal, and the cravings for unhealthy options slowly diminished as I embraced this new way of eating.

Another "don't" was overexertion. During the early stages of my journey, I had felt the need to push myself physically, thinking that by doing more, I would somehow accelerate my recovery. But this approach only led to burnout. My therapist stressed the importance of rest and gentle movements, explaining that healing required energy, and that overexertion could drain the body's reserves. I incorporated gentle stretching, short walks, and mindful breathing into my day, allowing my body to heal at its own pace rather than trying to force it into a schedule.

With time, these do's and don'ts became second nature. They served as both guidelines and reminders of the commitment I had made to myself. This structured approach was not restrictive; rather, it was empowering. Following these do's and don'ts gave me the sense that I was actively participating in my healing, making choices that honored my body and its needs.

Other Herbs

While *Cannabis sativa* and *CBD* had become cornerstones of my alternative treatment, they were only part of a broader spectrum of healing herbs. Each herb that my therapist introduced brought its unique properties to my regimen, addressing different aspects of my health and working synergistically to support my body's journey toward balance and vitality.

One of the key herbs was *Ashwagandha*, an adaptogen known for its ability to reduce stress and support the immune system. This herb became a nightly ritual, a gentle tea I sipped to calm my mind and prepare my body for rest. Ashwagandha worked to soothe my nervous system, countering the toll that months of anxiety and sleepless nights had taken. Over time, I noticed that my sleep improved, and with it, my energy levels during the day. This simple addition made a profound difference, helping me feel more grounded and resilient.

Another powerful herb was *Turmeric*, known for its anti-inflammatory and antioxidant properties. My therapist explained that chronic inflammation could hinder my body's healing process and contribute to pain, so I began incorporating turmeric into my meals and drinking it as tea. Paired with a pinch of black pepper to enhance its absorption, turmeric became a staple in my diet. I loved its earthy warmth, a daily reminder of the natural world's wisdom and the healing power of plants.

Ginger was also added to my regimen, particularly for its digestive and anti-inflammatory benefits. Not only did it aid in digestion, but it also provided relief from nausea, a lingering side effect of my chemotherapy sessions. Ginger became a comforting ally, a familiar taste that soothed my stomach and helped me feel more at ease. Whether grated into a tea or incorporated into my meals, ginger brought a sense of balance to my body, countering the residual effects of my previous treatments.

The most surprising addition was *Milk Thistle*, an herb revered for its ability to support liver health. Given the stress my body had endured with chemotherapy, my liver required support to process and eliminate toxins effectively. Milk Thistle became a daily supplement, a gentle but powerful tonic that aided in cleansing and restoring one of my body's essential organs. Over time, I began to feel lighter, as though my body was releasing the residual toxins and waste that had accumulated over the years of traditional treatments.

The integration of these herbs transformed my healing journey, providing my body with resources it needed to rebuild, restore, and thrive. Each herb brought its own form of nourishment and support, working in harmony with my body's natural rhythms. Together, they became a symphony of healing, a holistic approach that honored the complexity and resilience of my body.

Listening to My Body

One of the most profound lessons on this journey was learning to truly listen to my body. For years, I had relied on external voices—doctors, treatments, well-meaning friends—to tell me what was best for my health. But as I navigated this new path, I realized that my body had its own wisdom, a voice I had long ignored but could no longer afford to silence.

Listening to my body required patience and stillness. It meant pausing throughout the day to ask myself how I felt, tuning in to sensations of comfort or discomfort, energy or fatigue. There were days when my body craved rest, when every muscle ached for stillness. At first, it felt strange to indulge in these moments of quiet, as though I was betraying my instinct to "push through." But gradually, I began to see rest not as weakness but as a necessary act of love and respect for my healing.

This newfound awareness extended beyond rest. I began to notice how different foods made me feel, observing the effects they had on my energy and mood. When I ate whole, nourishing foods, my body responded with gratitude, rewarding me with strength and clarity. Conversely, when I veered from my regimen, choosing convenience over nourishment, I felt the effects almost immediately—a heaviness, a fogginess, a reminder that my body needed better fuel.

Listening to my body also meant honoring its signals, knowing when to stop or adjust if something didn't feel right. I learned that healing was not a linear process; it was filled with ebbs and flows, days of progress and moments of setback. In these moments, I reminded myself that healing was not a race. My body had endured years of hardship, and it deserved the time and space to heal on its own terms.

As I embraced this practice, I discovered an inner peace I hadn't felt in years. This process of listening, honoring, and responding to my body's needs became a form of meditation, a grounding ritual that reminded me of my strength and resilience. Through this deepened connection with myself, I realized that healing was not just a destination but a journey—one that I was learning to walk with grace, patience, and unwavering belief in my body's power to heal.

Chapter 7: Small Victories

Pain Relief

Pain had been a constant companion throughout my illness. It weighed on me, sometimes in sharp bursts, other times as a dull, relentless ache. My body felt foreign, a battlefield where each day brought a new threshold of discomfort. Yet, as I progressed in my alternative healing journey, I began noticing changes—small, nearly imperceptible at first, but they were there. These moments of reprieve marked the start of my small victories.

The first significant relief came as a surprise. After a particularly restful night, I woke up to find that the usual morning stiffness and aching joints were gone. I lay in bed, almost afraid to move, lest the pain return, but as I stretched and shifted, the discomfort that had been my constant companion was, for that morning, nowhere to be found. It was as if my body was whispering back to me, affirming that the path I'd chosen was beginning to work.

As days passed, these moments of relief grew more frequent. I celebrated each one, even if it was just an hour or two of diminished pain. I made notes in my journal, tracking these changes, reflecting on how far I had come. The herbs, diet, rest, and gentle movements were creating a balance within my body, easing inflammation, and allowing my system to recalibrate. Each pain-free moment became a victory that boosted my confidence and rekindled my hope.

One of the most challenging parts of healing had been managing the mental aspect of pain, and with relief, I found my mind was also beginning to relax. The fear of pain was receding, replaced by a growing faith in my body's ability to mend. My therapist reminded me often that the path to recovery was rarely linear and that setbacks might still happen, but my small victories built resilience within me, preparing me for whatever lay ahead.

Gradually, the fear began to lift. I learned to cherish these pain-free moments, however brief, as gifts, focusing on them rather than on the discomfort that often returned. In celebrating these victories, I found myself developing a deeper sense of gratitude—not only for the physical relief but for the reminder that healing was possible, even when progress came in small, fragile steps. These moments of pain relief were reminders that hope, too, could grow from the tiniest victories.

Moments of Joy

With the relief of pain came another unexpected gift: moments of pure, unfiltered joy. For so long, my focus had been on survival, on simply enduring each day without succumbing to despair. Now, as my body found pockets of relief, I found myself reconnecting with activities and feelings I had long set aside.

I remember one morning, sitting by the window with a cup of herbal tea, watching the sunrise. The colors were vibrant, a mixture of pinks, oranges, and purples painting the sky, and in that moment, I felt an overwhelming sense of peace. It wasn't happiness in the conventional sense; it was something quieter, something deeply rooted in the simple act of being present. The tea was warm in my hands, my body felt light, and for the first time in years, I felt an inexplicable joy.

These moments became a part of my day, little rituals of joy that sustained me. Some mornings, I would play soft music and let myself move, swaying gently to the rhythm, feeling my body respond with ease. Other times, I would read a book or look through old photo albums, letting nostalgia wash over me in waves. The images of past travels, family gatherings, and laughter-filled moments reminded me of who I was beyond the illness— a person who loved deeply, who found joy in the world around her.

My family became part of these joyful moments. Linda would join me for walks in the garden, pointing out blooming flowers or spotting birds in the trees. Jimmy, my youngest, would bring his crayons and drawings, proudly showing me his latest "masterpiece" as if it were a treasure of immeasurable value. Margaret would sit beside me and share stories from school, her laughter infectious, filling the room with a warmth that made my heart swell. Each of these moments was a small but powerful reminder of the life I was fighting for.

Even the simple act of preparing meals became a source of joy. I found comfort in chopping vegetables, stirring soups, and creating nourishing dishes for myself and my family. Cooking had always been therapeutic for me, and as I regained strength, I rediscovered the joy of creating food that was both healing and delicious. Each meal became a celebration of life, a testament to my resilience, and a reminder that joy could be found even in the smallest tasks.

As my health began to stabilize, my family sensed the shift and embraced these changes with open arms. They celebrated every milestone with me, their love and encouragement lighting the way. Even small achievements, like spending a whole day without pain or being able to walk a little farther than usual, were celebrated. We didn't need grand gestures; just being together, sharing these quiet victories, was enough.

One evening, as the holidays approached, Albert gathered the kids and surprised me with an early Christmas celebration. The house was adorned with lights and decorations, their warm glow filling our home with a sense of festivity that I hadn't felt in years. My daughters had strung lights around the windows, and Jimmy insisted on placing ornaments on every available surface. The house was alive with laughter, and I felt surrounded by love.

That evening, as we gathered around the dinner table, my family presented me with a small cake, decorated with a single candle. They encouraged me to make a wish. Closing my eyes, I felt a surge of emotion—gratitude, hope, love—and I wished for the strength to continue on this path, to keep finding healing in each day. The room was silent for a moment as I blew out the candle, and then cheers erupted around me, their joyful faces reflecting the love that had carried me through my darkest days.

Family celebrations became a regular part of our lives. Each week, we would find a reason to gather together, sometimes for a shared meal, other times just to sit together and talk.

These celebrations were a way of honoring our journey, of marking the milestones and victories, no matter how small. My family had been my anchor, grounding me in love and joy, reminding me of the beauty in togetherness.

Over time, these family gatherings became a tradition. We found solace in our shared moments, knowing that no matter what the future held, we had each other. My illness had tested us, but it had also brought us closer, reminding us of the fragility of life and the importance of cherishing every moment. These celebrations were more than just gatherings; they were acts of resilience, a testament to the power of love to heal, to uplift, and to transform.

In the end, it was these small victories—relief from pain, moments of joy, and the strength of my family—that became the building blocks of my healing journey. They reminded me that while healing was a long road, it was paved with love, joy, and the unwavering support of those who walked beside me.

Chapter 8: Laughter, Love, and Lightness

Cancer has a way of altering your perspective on life, forcing you to face some of the most difficult realities with strength, resilience, and sometimes, humor. When I first received my diagnosis, the weight of it all felt unbearable. The treatments, the pain, and the emotional toll seemed insurmountable. But as I went through the process, I learned an essential lesson: laughter was a balm for the soul.

At first, I wasn't sure if I could laugh again. I had been so consumed by my illness that the idea of finding humor in anything felt foreign. But little by little, I realized that laughter could coexist with suffering. It didn't erase the pain or the challenges, but it made the journey more bearable.

I remember one particularly rough day during chemotherapy when I felt physically drained and emotionally empty. As I lay in bed, trying to muster the strength to get through another day, my husband Albert walked into the room. He had an uncanny ability to lighten any situation, and on that day, he decided to put on a silly hat he had found at a thrift store. It was a giant, purple, feathered monstrosity that made him look like a clown. His attempt to cheer me up was nothing short of absurd, but in that moment, I couldn't help but laugh. The ridiculousness of the situation broke the heaviness that had settled in my heart. Albert's laughter was infectious, and soon I was laughing so hard, I could barely catch my breath.

That moment of humor became a turning point for me. It reminded me that even in the darkest times, humor could be a source of healing. Laughter didn't mean I was denying my reality—it meant I was giving myself permission to experience joy even amidst suffering. I started looking for opportunities to laugh every day, even if it was just a silly joke from a friend or a funny TV show that distracted me from the pain. Slowly, I began to see humor as a tool to regain control over my mind, a way to resist letting the disease consume me entirely.

Albert was always my partner in finding humor. We would joke about my chemotherapy treatments and laugh at the most trivial things. He would often crack jokes about the weird foods I had to eat during my healing process, making fun of my strange concoctions of herbal teas and bizarre diets. He turned my restrictions into comedy, and somehow, it made it all easier to accept. I realized that laughter wasn't just a temporary distraction—it was a form of resistance. It was a defiance against the disease, a way of saying, "You may have my body, but you'll never have my spirit."

As the treatments continued, humor became a coping mechanism, a way of confronting the harsh realities of illness with a light heart. It gave me permission to not take everything so seriously, to embrace the absurdity of life, and to find moments of joy in the most unexpected places. I found strength in laughter, and that strength helped me push forward, even when the road was difficult.

Family Fun

The healing process is not just about physical recovery—it's also about emotional and mental restoration. And for me, the healing power of family fun became an essential part of my journey. During my illness, I realized that my family was my greatest source of joy. Their love, support, and the simple moments we shared together were invaluable.

Linda, Margaret, and Jimmy each found their own ways to make me smile. When I was too weak to go out, they would come up with creative ways to bring the world to me. Linda, my eldest, loved to bake, and one of her favorite pastimes was trying out new cookie recipes. She would set up a mini "cookie factory" in the kitchen, where she and her sisters would make a mess, and I would sit back and watch them. The smell of fresh-baked cookies would fill the house, and even though I couldn't eat much, I felt content just to be surrounded by the chaos and joy of it all.

Jimmy, with his endless energy, was always the entertainer. He would run around the house, creating imaginary worlds and insisting that I be the "queen" of his kingdom. His innocent humor was a reminder of the pure joy that still existed in the world. He would make funny faces or tell silly jokes, and I would laugh, even if it was just for a moment. That laughter, coming from the heart of a seven-year-old, reminded me of the beauty in simplicity—the ability to find joy in the smallest of things.

Margaret, my quiet, thoughtful daughter, would often sit with me in the evenings and tell me stories or ask me about the past. Her inquisitive nature was a gift, and as we laughed over silly memories or made fun of the things I had done as a teenager, I felt a deep sense of connection to her. Even when we weren't laughing, just being in each other's company brought a sense of peace.

We also found ways to bond through games. There were nights when we would pull out old board games and have family competitions. I'll never forget the night we played charades, where Albert's wild gestures had us all in stitches. I had forgotten how much fun we could have together, and those moments of laughter helped us navigate the difficulty of my illness.

Family fun didn't have to be extravagant; it didn't require expensive outings or grand gestures. Sometimes, it was just about being present with each other, making the best of what we had. It was about finding joy in the simple moments and letting that joy heal us, piece by piece.

Light in the Darkness

Cancer has a way of casting long shadows, and there were times when I felt overwhelmed by the weight of it all. The pain, the treatments, the uncertainty of the future—it all seemed like too much to bear. But even in the darkest moments, I found light in unexpected places. That light often came from the people around me, from the love and support of my family, and from within myself.

The darkest days were often the ones when I felt the most alone. There were nights when the pain was unbearable, and I would lie in bed, wondering if I would ever feel "normal" again. But then, in the midst of that darkness, something would shift. It could be a message from a friend, a phone call from a loved one, or a quiet moment of reflection. I began to realize that even in my darkest hours, I wasn't truly alone. The love of my family and the support of those who cared for me became a constant source of light.

One of the most profound moments of light came when I least expected it. I had been feeling especially low, overwhelmed by the toll cancer had taken on my body and my spirit. But one evening, as I sat with Albert, he took my hand and reminded me of all the battles we had fought together—of all the times we had overcome adversity. His words, simple but filled with conviction, were like a light shining through the darkness.

"I'm with you," he said. "We're in this together."

It was in that moment that I understood what true healing was. It wasn't just about overcoming cancer—it was about facing the darkness with love, with laughter, and with light. It was about knowing that even in the hardest times, there was still a glimmer of hope, a way forward.

The more I embraced that light, the more it grew. I began to see the world differently—not as a place of suffering, but as one filled with possibilities. I learned that even the darkest days had something to offer, something to teach me. Those moments of light became my guiding stars, reminding me that no matter how hard the journey, there was always a way through it.

In the end, it wasn't just the absence of pain or the disappearance of illness that marked my healing—it was the ability to find light in the darkness. The laughter, the love, and the lightness that I found in those moments of adversity became the foundation of my recovery. They were the fuel that kept me going, the strength that helped me push through, and the reminder that, no matter how difficult the road, there was always hope.

Chapter 9: Tested and Trusted Therapies

Therapies That Worked

When I first began my journey with cervical cancer, the overwhelming number of treatment options left me feeling more confused than confident. I was bombarded with medical advice, alternative therapies, and countless recommendations from well-meaning friends and family. Every doctor, every healer, every patient seemed to have a different approach, and it was a challenge to find the one that would actually help me. However, through trial and error, research, and a deep trust in my own intuition, I found therapies that truly worked—both physically and emotionally.

The conventional treatments I underwent, particularly chemotherapy and radiation, were necessary and powerful in shrinking the tumors and eliminating cancer cells. However, these treatments came with an arsenal of harsh side effects: nausea, fatigue, hair loss, and the emotional toll of seeing my body change. The physical pain was one thing, but the emotional pain of feeling "less than" was almost as difficult to bear. Despite this, chemotherapy worked to eradicate the cancer from my system, and it was crucial in my fight for survival.

But conventional medicine was not the whole story. During my treatment journey, I came across therapies that complemented the harsh medical treatments and provided relief in ways I hadn't anticipated. One of the most beneficial was the use of cannabis sativa and cannabidiol (CBD). Cannabis had always been a controversial topic, but my decision to incorporate it into my healing regimen came after speaking with a doctor who specialized in integrative medicine. I started using a CBD oil tincture to alleviate my chronic pain and anxiety. The results were nothing short of transformative. CBD helped reduce my pain levels, improved my sleep, and alleviated much of the nausea caused by chemotherapy. It also had a calming effect on my anxiety, something I hadn't expected but greatly appreciated as my mental health was just as important as my physical health in this journey.

Alongside the use of cannabis, I incorporated herbal therapies like ginger, turmeric, and milk thistle. Ginger tea became a regular part of my daily routine. It helped with my digestive issues, soothed my stomach after treatments, and had anti-inflammatory properties that supported my body during the healing process.

Turmeric, with its high levels of curcumin, acted as a potent anti-inflammatory, further helping my body recover from the inflammation caused by both the cancer and the treatments. Milk thistle was suggested to me by a holistic nutritionist to support liver function. Given the toxicity of the chemotherapy drugs, this herb became vital in helping my liver process and eliminate the toxins that were building up.

Another important part of my regimen was the acupuncture treatments I started after reading about their efficacy in supporting cancer patients. Acupuncture worked wonders in reducing the pain from radiation and chemotherapy, but perhaps more importantly, it helped to balance my energy levels. The calming effect it had on me allowed me to approach the healing process from a place of mindfulness and relaxation. I found that my body became more receptive to healing when I gave it space to relax and heal energetically.

The combination of these therapies, both traditional and alternative, brought me much-needed relief and made the process of healing more manageable. It wasn't about relying on just one treatment; it was about finding the right combination for me. Everyone's journey is different, but for me, integrating cannabis, herbal remedies, acupuncture, and mindfulness created the healing environment I needed to move forward.

Self-Care and Wellness

As I embarked on the path of recovery, one of the most profound lessons I learned was the importance of self-care. In the beginning, I was so focused on fighting the cancer that I neglected my own needs. I didn't recognize how vital it was to take care of my body, mind, and spirit during this challenging time. The stress of chemotherapy, doctor's appointments, and trying to maintain some semblance of a normal life took a toll on me. It wasn't until I slowed down and embraced the concept of self-care that I began to feel better, both mentally and physically.

Self-care is not just about pampering yourself with spa days or indulgent treats—though those moments do help—it's about learning how to listen to your body, give yourself permission to rest, and treat yourself with the kindness and compassion you deserve. This became especially important for me during my recovery. There were days when I was physically exhausted, and rather than pushing through or ignoring my body's signals, I learned to honor them. I started to give myself the gift of rest, listening to my body's cues rather than forcing myself to "power through" like I had always done in the past.

I learned the importance of eating well. Throughout my treatments, I focused on nourishing my body with nutrient-dense foods. I made sure to incorporate a wide variety of fruits, vegetables, and whole grains into my diet, focusing on foods that were anti-inflammatory and detoxifying. I paid special attention to anti-cancer foods, such as berries, cruciferous vegetables like broccoli and kale, and green tea. I also began drinking fresh vegetable juices every morning to support my immune system and keep my energy levels stable.

Hydration was another key component of my self-care. I used to overlook the importance of water in my daily life, but I soon realized that staying hydrated was essential for supporting my immune system and flushing out toxins from the chemotherapy. Every morning, I made a point to start my day with a glass of water and continued drinking throughout the day.

In addition to physical self-care, I recognized the importance of mental and emotional wellness. I began practicing meditation and mindfulness daily. Meditation helped me manage the anxiety that came with uncertainty, and it became a safe space where I could reconnect with my inner peace. It was through meditation that I realized I had to let go of fear. I started to embrace the notion that healing was a process, and that I didn't have to have all the answers right away. Allowing myself to feel my emotions without judgment—whether it was fear, sadness, or anger—was liberating. It made me feel more in control of my healing journey.

I also surrounded myself with positive energy—people who supported me and uplifted me. My family and friends were my support network, but I also connected with others going through similar experiences. Support groups, both online and in person, allowed me to share my journey with others and hear theirs. It reminded me that I wasn't alone, and that there were many paths to healing. The connection with others was a form of healing in itself, as it provided emotional validation and shared strength.

By prioritizing self-care, I was able to balance the demands of my cancer treatment while also honoring my body, mind, and spirit. Self-care became a cornerstone of my recovery, and I learned that it wasn't selfish to focus on myself—it was necessary for my healing.

One of the most important things I've learned through my journey is that knowledge is power. When I was first diagnosed, I was overwhelmed with the medical jargon and the uncertainty of the road ahead. However, as I began researching, speaking with doctors, and connecting with others who had been through similar experiences, I gained the knowledge I needed to make informed decisions about my treatment. Cancer doesn't discriminate, and every survivor has their own unique story. But there are key lessons that can help others facing the same battle.

The first lesson I would impart to others is to trust your body. It's easy to get lost in the world of medical advice, to feel overwhelmed by the myriad of treatments and therapies available. But your body is the ultimate guide. If something doesn't feel right or you have concerns about a treatment plan, speak up. Advocate for yourself. In my case, this meant asking questions about every therapy, whether conventional or alternative, before agreeing to it. It meant being open to trying new things but also being discerning and trusting my instincts when something didn't sit well with me.

Another piece of advice I would give is to be proactive in your healing. You are not just a passive recipient of treatment; you are an active participant in your own recovery. Learn about the therapies available to you, both traditional and alternative. Explore complementary treatments, but also be sure to discuss them with your oncologist. Some therapies, like acupuncture or CBD, can enhance the effectiveness of conventional treatments, but others may not be suitable for everyone. Having a team of medical professionals who support your holistic approach is essential.

Don't be afraid to embrace alternative therapies. While they shouldn't replace medical treatment, they can offer invaluable support. I found that incorporating herbal therapies, acupuncture, and mindfulness practices helped reduce my symptoms, alleviate my stress, and improve my quality of life. These therapies supported my body in ways that made the more traditional treatments easier to handle. Cannabis, for instance, wasn't just a pain reliever—it gave me a sense of mental clarity and peace that I hadn't felt in months.

Finally, I would encourage cancer fighters to lean on your support network. It's easy to feel isolated in this fight, but you don't have to go through it alone. Reach out to family, friends, support groups, and counselors. Your journey may be personal, but the strength and love of those around you can make all the difference.

As I share my story, I hope that others facing similar battles can draw strength from my experience. There is no one-size-fits-all solution to cancer treatment, but through knowledge, self-care, and the courage to try new therapies, healing is possible. We are all warriors in this fight, and the knowledge we gain along the way can empower us to win.

Chapter 10: Christmas Bliss

Christmas had always been a time of joy and celebration, but that year, it took on a deeper, more profound meaning. After everything I had been through—diagnosis, treatments, the emotional rollercoaster—it was hard to believe that I was now here, on the other side, celebrating another Christmas. In a sense, this holiday marked my rebirth, my renewal. It was a time when I could fully appreciate the moments I used to take for granted.

The process of healing wasn't just about physical recovery; it was about reconnecting with myself and rediscovering the simple joys in life. And in the midst of that rediscovery, Christmas became the ultimate celebration of my survival. I had learned to savor life in ways

I never had before, and the holiday season only magnified that newfound appreciation.

As I reflected on the past year, I couldn't help but feel an overwhelming sense of gratitude. Gratitude for the doctors and medical professionals who helped me along the way. Gratitude for the natural therapies that had eased my pain, soothed my spirit, and supported my healing. But more than anything, I felt gratitude for my family. They had been my unwavering source of support, love, and strength, especially in those moments when I felt weak or hopeless. The sense of community and love they provided me through this journey was immeasurable.

Gratitude was a transformative emotion, and I began to understand how essential it was for healing. It wasn't just about being thankful for the good moments, but also for the tough ones.

The difficult days, the tears, the fears—they had shaped me into a stronger, more resilient person. And as I sat in front of the Christmas tree, the twinkling lights reflecting in my eyes, I realized that it wasn't just about surviving cancer; it was about being truly alive.

The holidays also allowed me to look beyond myself and acknowledge the collective strength of those who had supported me, and those who were fighting their own battles. In every ornament on the tree, every carol sung, I saw a reminder of the love and resilience that could carry us through even the darkest times. It was a heart full of gratitude that allowed me to see the beauty in life, even in the moments that felt broken.

What struck me the most was how healing gratitude could be. The simple act of being thankful for what I had, instead of dwelling on what I had lost, was powerful. It helped me reframe my narrative. Cancer had altered my life, yes, but it hadn't defined me. The support I received, the love I felt, and the strength I had cultivated all gave me a new perspective on what truly mattered. Gratitude, I realized, was not just a feeling—it was a practice, a mindset, and a gift that I could carry with me long after Christmas.

As we celebrated that Christmas, I marveled at the beauty of how far I had come. The love of my family, the peace of mind I had found through my healing journey, and the joy of being surrounded by those I held most dear were the greatest gifts I could have ever received. My heart was full, and that fullness gave me the energy to keep moving forward. There was still so much to be done, but in that moment, I was simply thankful for this breath, this life, and all the possibilities that still lay ahead.

Christmas had always been a time of joy in our home, but this year, it felt like we were celebrating on a deeper level, one that transcended the typical holiday cheer. After my cancer journey, Christmas became not just a seasonal celebration but a profound celebration of life itself. This was a time when we could honor the moments we often take for granted—being together, being healthy, and being able to cherish each other. After everything I had gone through, I learned that the real gift of Christmas wasn't the presents under the tree or the grand feasts; it was the simple act of being alive to experience it all.

Our home, which had once felt quiet and subdued during the months of my treatments, was now filled with the joyful chaos that accompanies a Christmas celebration. The tree sparkled in the corner of the living room, the sweet smell of cinnamon and pine wafted through the air, and laughter echoed off the walls as my children excitedly prepared for the holiday festivities. We baked cookies together, hung stockings with care, and shared stories of past Christmases. It was a renewal of the traditions that had been put on hold during my darkest days.

What made this year's celebration unique was the deep meaning behind every moment. We had come through a significant trial, and now, we could enjoy Christmas in a way that felt like a true victory. I didn't need extravagant gifts or lavish celebrations. What mattered was the shared experience of being together—of my children seeing me healthier, of my husband and I laughing again, and of all of us being reminded of the beauty in the smallest moments.

In the lead-up to Christmas Eve, I felt a surge of peace. In the past, the holiday season often came with a rush to finish shopping, to prepare extravagant meals, and to meet social obligations. But that year, I had shed all the unnecessary stress. I didn't feel pressured to put on a perfect show for anyone. Instead, I focused on the things that truly mattered: time spent with loved ones, meaningful conversations, and quiet moments of reflection. There was no need to rush around; I embraced the serenity of slowing down and truly soaking in the beauty of the season.

The most powerful part of the Christmas celebration was the gratitude that underpinned every moment. We expressed our thanks for each other, for the ability to celebrate, and for the strength we had shown through the previous year. This wasn't just another Christmas—it was a Christmas that marked the triumph of life over illness, the victory of love over fear. There was an unspoken sense of renewal in the air, as if the holiday itself was a metaphor for my journey: from darkness to light, from struggle to peace, from illness to wellness.

That Christmas was a sacred time, a chance for me to look back on everything I had overcome and forward to everything that was yet to come. It felt like the closing of one chapter and the beginning of a new one. As I looked around the room at my family, I realized that this was the true meaning of Christmas—a celebration of life, love, and the power of resilience. We were not just marking the season; we were celebrating a new chapter in our lives, one in which we had triumphed together.

Hope for Others

As the Christmas season drew to a close, I couldn't help but think of the many others who were still in the midst of their cancer battles. While I was fortunate enough to be celebrating with my family, I knew that many were still facing the uncertainty, pain, and fear that cancer brings. I had been given a second chance, and that gift made me feel an overwhelming sense of responsibility to share my story, my healing journey, and the lessons I had learned along the way with others.

It became clear to me that part of my healing process was to use my experience to bring hope to those who needed it most. I had lived through the darkest days of my life, and now I had the ability to offer light to others. I thought about the countless cancer patients who were struggling to find peace in the midst of their pain, who were uncertain about their prognosis, who felt hopeless. I wanted them to know that healing was possible, that there were therapies that worked, and that hope was always worth holding on to, no matter how dire things seemed.

Hope, I realized, was the foundation of every healing journey. Without hope, we have nothing. But hope wasn't just about wishing for a miracle. It was about being proactive, seeking out solutions, and creating a mindset of **possibility** rather than one of defeat. The therapies I used to heal—from chemotherapy to cannabis to mindfulness—had each played a role in building my hope, as had the support of my family and the strength I found within myself.

As I reflected on what had worked for me, I decided to share that knowledge with others. I started writing about my journey, speaking at local support groups, and reaching out to people in my community who were struggling with cancer. The more I shared, the more I realized that there was power in telling our stories. When we speak our truths, we give others the courage to do the same. And through that sharing, we build a network of support that can carry us through the darkest times.

My Christmas wish that year was not just for my own continued health—it was for hope for others. I wanted those who were still fighting to feel empowered, to find peace, and to know that they were not alone in their battle. I wanted to help them believe that a future full of joy and possibility was possible, just as I had believed for myself when I couldn't see the way forward.

Christmas had given me the gift of gratitude, and now it was time for me to give the gift of hope to others. This season wasn't just about celebrating my own survival; it was about helping others find their way through the darkness and into the light. Together, we could heal, together, we could find joy, and together, we could hold onto the hope that would see us through.

Afterword

As I close this chapter of my life and this book, I am filled with an overwhelming sense of gratitude, reflection, and hope. This journey, from my diagnosis to healing, has been nothing short of transformative. It has been a journey of resilience, of faith, of love, and ultimately, of finding light in the most unexpected of places. The lessons I've learned through this experience are lessons I will carry with me for the rest of my life.

When I first received the news of my diagnosis, I felt as though the world had come crashing down around me. It was a moment of disbelief, a moment when time seemed to stand still. But what followed that diagnosis was not just the physical battle of cancer, but a deeper, more profound struggle—the fight for my spirit. How does one maintain hope when the future is uncertain? How does one hold onto joy when pain and fear seem to be the only companions? It was a journey of learning to trust again—in my body, in my healing, and in the people around me.

Through the course of this book, I've shared the raw, honest experiences of what it meant to fight cancer—not just through medical treatments, but also through the emotional, mental, and spiritual battles that came with it. Every chapter of this book represents not just a moment of survival, but a testament to the power of the human spirit. It is a reflection of how healing is not just about the absence of illness, but about the restoration of hope, the rebuilding of relationships, and the embrace of life itself.

One of the most important aspects of this journey was discovering the importance of self-care—of listening to my body, of seeking out healing methods that resonated with me, and of being open to the idea that there are alternative therapies that can complement traditional medicine. My exploration of natural remedies, mindfulness, and therapies like cannabis and cannabidiol helped me regain control over my body and emotions. It taught me that healing is not one-size-fits-all; it is a deeply personal experience that requires patience, faith, and an openness to what works for you.

But even beyond the therapies, this book is about the incredible support system that surrounded me. It's about the strength of my family, the love of my friends, and the unwavering belief in me from those who walked beside me during my darkest days. Cancer is not a solitary fight—it's one that involves the support of others, the hands that lift you when you can't stand on your own, and the hearts that carry you when your own feels too heavy. I dedicate this book to every person who has been part of my journey, and to all those who are still walking their own paths toward healing.

The greatest gift I received throughout this process was the gift of perspective. Cancer has a way of forcing you to see life through a different lens. You begin to appreciate the moments that once seemed trivial, like the sound of your children's laughter, the feel of sunlight on your face, and the simple joy of being surrounded by the people you love. It forces you to embrace gratitude in its purest form. For me, it was the realization that life is fragile, and that the time we have should be cherished—not just for the big moments, but for the quiet, everyday moments that bring us true happiness.

As I reflect on the pages of this book, I am reminded that healing is a journey—one that doesn't have a specific end date or final destination. It is a continuous process of growth, of learning to trust ourselves and our bodies again, of seeking peace, and of finding joy in the most unexpected of places. I may never be the same person I was before my diagnosis, but I am stronger, wiser, and more appreciative of the life I now have. And I am hopeful—hopeful that my journey can offer encouragement to others who may find themselves walking a similar path.

This book is not just my story. It is the story of anyone who has ever faced illness, loss, or adversity and found the strength to keep moving forward. It is a story of hope, resilience, and the unwavering belief that healing is possible, no matter how difficult the road may seem. It is a reminder that we are not defined by our circumstances, but by how we rise above them.

To anyone who is currently fighting cancer, or any illness for that matter, I want you to know that you are not alone. Your journey is valid, your pain is real, but there is always hope. There are always new options to explore, new therapies to try, and new ways to heal. I hope that my story can serve as a source of inspiration, and that you can find the strength to continue fighting, day by day, no matter how difficult the road may seem.

To those who are supporting a loved one through illness, I hope you recognize the power of your presence. Your love, your support, and your belief in your loved one are immeasurable gifts. You are part of the healing process in ways you may not even realize. Continue to show up, to be present, and to offer compassion, because your strength is a lifeline.

Finally, as I sit here today, healthy and hopeful, I look forward to the future with a heart full of gratitude, a spirit full of joy, and a life full of possibility. This Christmas, I celebrated not just the season, but the life I had fought for. And I carry with me the hope that anyone who reads this book will understand that healing is a journey worth taking, no matter how long it takes.

Thank you for being part of my journey. Thank you for reading my story. And most importantly, thank you for believing in the power of **hope, love, and resilience**. The greatest gift of all is that we can continue to heal, continue to grow, and continue to live with purpose, no matter what challenges come our way.

With all my love and gratitude,

Laura McGregor

www.ingramcontent.com/pod-product-compliance
Lightning Source LLC
Chambersburg PA
CBHW071010250726

48653CB00005B/1575